EAST & WEST

by

M.J. Cunningham

and

I-Yen Yang, M.D.

Acupuncture:
An
Alternative to Suffering

FIRST EDITION

Library of Congress Catalog Card No: 93-93901
ISBN: 1-56002-340-6

UNIVERSITY EDITIONS, Inc.
59 Oak Lane, Spring Valley
Huntington, West Virginia 25704

Cover by Cindy Schubert

Dedication

To a special man, a special doctor, I-Yen Yang for his invaluable assistance and encouragement. Also to a very special lady named Virginia, who should be an inspiration to us all.

This book was written for all of you who suffer in silence, enduring your pain and suffering, not knowing there is help and hope for all of you through Acupuncture treatments. Bless you all.

Table of Contents

Foreword

This book could have and should have been finished some time ago, but friends, family and people who know it is being written, keep asking me about Acupuncture treatment only the doctor can answer. He is a very busy man taking care of many patients, so calling him for answers to pertinent questions like, "Why does the doctor put a needle in the back of your leg for back pain?" and "Why does he put a needle in the back of your neck to stop a headache in the front of your head?" "Why does the doctor put a needle in your left leg when the pain is in your right leg and hip?" On and on the questions keep coming, but I don't have the answers, only the doctor does. He treats me, I get relief, have more energy, that's all I need to know, it works! There will be a few diagrams in this book for you, but if you are like me, you won't understand any more about how Acupuncture works than the rest of us.

One question keeps coming up, week after week from people who NEED an answer to a very important question. "What about AIDS? and the use of all the needles? Does the doctor throw away the needles he uses on each patient?" "What if someone is HIV positive but doesn't tell the doctor before treatment?" Today I asked Doctor Yang these questions. He told me he uses an "Autoclave", which is another word for sterilizer. A machine in which he puts in sterile water, puts down the lid, turns on the power, the water makes steam and the needles are sterilized. He also uses chlorine or alcohol in vials. Doctor said he has a great many needles, so no one need be concerned about, "catching anything" from the use of the needles.

There are some practitioners of Acupuncture who use disposable needles, but they are not all (if any) medical doctors. Personally, I prefer an M.D.

Dr. Yang is certified by the American Board of Internal Medicine and each sub-specialty board.

Dr. Yang is also a Doctor of Oncology, Hematology, Immunology and Internal Medicine. I am sure he knows what is best for his patients.

—M.J. Cunningham

Preface

This book was written out of my true desire to help other people to know there is an alterative to pain and many other problems Western medicine can not, or will not be able to cure through ordinary Western medical technology. This insatiable desire to get the message out to anyone who will read it, has been with me for many years. Now it is done. I am grateful to Doctor Yang who, without his technical knowledge and help, it would never have been written.

—M.J. Cunningham
Umatilla, OR.
October, 1992

Chapter 1

My First Encounter With Acupuncture

My first encounter with Sciatica, was when I was in premedical school. One of my classmates and I joined the Judo Club as extracurricular activity. My classmate sustained a backache first, then later had to have a surgical procedure done, with favorable results. I sustained backache, not at the time of the Judo lesson, but later when I tried to straighten my back while walking along the street.

Rather than taking me to the family doctor, my mother took me to see a "Gong Fu Master" who scared me with the possibility of an atrophic change of the affected leg in the future. "A drumstick knee," was how he put it. The back pain was relieved spontaneously in time, and no atrophy ever happened to my leg to date.

During my residency training, the medical journals frequently talked about the serious consequence of Sciatic involvement. The trend of thinking has turned around since, and a more conservative approach becomes the mainstream of thinking. The exceptions being, loss of muscle power and or dysfunction of the Viscera. Even then, Acupuncture may work.

Occasionally, a patient with sciatica will have bowel and urinary symptoms which can be cured by treating the back pain.

All the symptoms will improve with the treatment to the back according to my experience. Since all the nerve endings contribute to the lower back, and also distribute to the pelvic area, this can be a source of confusion in the female patient. Careful history taking and a physical examination usually identify the real cause, and proper treatment of the back relieves the symptoms.

A case in point: A 58 year old man came to see me not knowing if I could help him or not. He had had an operation for cancer of the rectum in 1987. He received 5 weeks of radiation treatments and a year of fluorouracil. Since then he has had gas all the time with, leakage of the stool at times. A year ago a diagnosis of radiation colitis was given. For the past several months impotence became a problem; insufficient erection. He told me he has had chronic lower back pain off and on since the age of 17, after a bad fall which has left him with right sciatica. This man has been to chiropractors in the past. He was given a treatment with success with bowels, and back pain diminished. Five months later he returned much better and very pleased with his progress. Further treatment of 6 or more sessions were only to strengthen the conclusion of continued improvement.

—I-Yen Yang, M.D.

Chapter 2

Acupuncture, An Alternative To Pain

This is a book I have wanted to write for twenty years, ever since my first experience with Acupuncture.

I had a serious accident in which, slipping and falling on a wet concrete porch, bouncing down five concrete steps on my rear and right hip, managed to knock myself out with a broken hip and right leg. No one seemed to notice me laying in a lump at the bottom of the stairs, for what seemed like forever. Finally, someone noticed and summoned help. You know what? You really do see colored stars, just before you go out.

After a long period of hospital stays, the use of my legs was gone. Not being able to walk, using a wheelchair to get around in and sleeping in a hospital bed at home, I was taken back to the hospital, only to be told by one of the best orthopedic surgeons around, (he was a dear friend by now) "There is nothing more we can do for you, I am going to send you to a doctor of Acupuncture". My reply was, "Thank God".

I was happy to be sent to (I will call him Dr. Smith) knowing if there was a chance for me to ever walk again, it would be through him and Acupuncture treatments.

As you know, pain is the hardest and most dominant of our senses to deal with.

It is not only hard for us to deal with, but our families suffer too. We don't feel like we used to, we don't think like we did, so our families and friends think they should be able to help us feel useful and happy. Well, we try to stay happy and appear to enjoy their efforts but when they feel they can no longer be of help they start to drift away, feeling guilty that they can't stop the pain and our feelings of frustration. Can't blame them. We lay or sit there trying to focus on their conversation, half drugged with pain killers and wishing they would go, so we can sink into drugged sleep or some kind of relief.

I was not able to have surgery to correct or fix what was wrong with my back because I am allergic to the dye used in an Angiogram, so it was pain shots, cortisone shots, physical therapy, and traction for me. It seemed there was no help for me until I was sent for Acupuncture.

When people heard I was going for Acupuncture treatments years ago, they thought it was some kind of weird "stuff" used only in China, if they even knew where it came from, and couldn't believe it would work on "WHITE" people. Let me tell you how well it worked on this "WHITE" person.

Being driven to and carried into the doctors' office with the greatest of hopes of walking again, I had had in almost three years, I was put in a quiet darkened room with soft peaceful music drifting in.

Lying there trying to relax, I waited for what I thought would be a giant of a man in a white coat, but in walked a man who looked like John Denver, wire rimmed glasses and all. He introduced himself, and in a soft voice asked me if I had any experience with Acupuncture or even knew how it worked. Remember I was in a lot of pain and didn't feel much like talking, but he made me feel so much at ease, hope filled me.

After three treatments three times a week for three weeks, I was able to stand on my own and slide one foot in front of the other for a short distance down the hall. Please remember, I was bedridden and not even able to stand, so this seemed like a Miracle to me and those who had watched as I was carried in and out of the office three times a week. My doctor and two nurses had tears in their eyes, and were clapping their hands as if they were witnessing a miracle. To me it was.

Continuing treatments for nearly a year, I was able to run, dance, and swim again, not to mention being able to play with my little girl. She had just turned one year old when I fell. It seems funny now, but she really thought the hospital was one of our homes because, "Mommie" spent so much time there.

Maybe one has to give up all hope of western medicine helping or healing them before trying Acupuncture, maybe not. Maybe it is like hitting bottom, before you can climb up with hope in your heart, and a strong will to stand on your own two feet again. To fight back when you are told there is no hope, to believe in your doctors' ability to make the right decisions for you.

There was one time in my life of pain when I wanted to give up, to die, if I had to be pushed around in a wheelchair and be a burden. To me, being sent to a doctor of Acupuncture was the beginning of life itself.

Being a short, redheaded freckled faced girl growing up on a horse ranch, I learned to fight for just about everything that meant anything to me.

Being a fighter, being bedridden was not for me or my family. Maybe being a sickly kid, overcoming that, going on to be a dancer, iceskater, gymnast and a baseball player, it was not in me to give up.

Twenty years and three accidents later, I am back with a great doctor of Acupuncture, who is one of the best.

Wanting to write this book for so long, so others who might read it, will know there is an alternative to pain, allergies, Chronic-Fatigue-Syndrome, asthma, you name it, it can be cured or at least greatly helped. Maybe you need a little more faith in your body's ability to heal it's self with the help of Acupuncture. I don't know, all I can tell you is, there is light at the end of the tunnel.

Acupuncture has worked for me and continues to help me to help others.

My doctor is good, but there are

others out there to help you. Be sure to look around and get an M.D. Don't give up hope because, life is wonderful when you feel good.

You have been good enough to read this far about my experiences with Acupuncture, now I would like to tell you about a lady I met, quite by accident.

Chapter 3

Don't Give Up

While at the library, a lady began talking to me about the way the restroom was designed. We laughed about it, then she just started talking, the way we women do, and it seems she has had a problem with hemorrhaging for years, with no relief given to her by all the specialists she has seen through the years. This lady has given up all hope of ever being cured and has given up on life. She was talking about, "ending it all", because she felt lost, alone, and tired of going to doctors only to be told there was no hope of a cure.

You might think this was some old wasted lady but, she was in her early forties, with a degree in engineering and also has a teaching degree. What a waste of life and brains. I asked if she had considered Acupuncture as an alternative to Western medicine, she said, "no". "Will you please see my doctor, I know he can help you", I asked? She said she would think about it. The next week when I went in for treatment, I asked my doctor if she had come in, he said, "NO". Maybe she will show up yet. It took me two years to make an appointment with doctor Yang and I KNEW better.

Dr. Yang has many degrees and specialties too numerous to mention here, but we will get into some of his case histories as we go along.

Chapter 4

Questions People Ask

The questions most people ask me when they know I have taken Acupuncture treatments are: "does it hurt?" "does it work?" and, "how long does it take to work?" Not once has anyone asked if it was expensive.

Expense doesn't seem to be the main concern of relief from pain. NO, it does not hurt. The needles are as fine as a coarse hair from a head of hair. Some are short, others are longer. There seem to be several sizes for different parts of the body and seasons of the year. "Seasons of the year"? you might ask. Yes, different times of the year affect the depth the needle is gently twirled into the skin, fat, and muscle. Skin deep, in the Spring; Subcutaneous tissue, in the Summer; muscle, in the Fall; bone and sinew, in the winter.

Now, can you picture in your mind a clock or pie plate, or anything flat and round? Now if you can see this cut into 12 pieces, like pieces of pie, starting at 12 o'clock, this is where the Acuflow starts at 3 a.m. with the lung Acuflow, reaches the Colon at 5 a.m., the Stomach at 7 a.m., Spleen at 9 a.m., Heart at 11 a.m., the Intestines at 1 p.m., the Bladder at 3 p.m., the Kidneys at 5 p.m., the Cardiover at 7 p.m., Trifoci at 9 p.m., Gallbladder at 11 p.m., the Liver at 1 a.m., and finally moves through Liver Acuflow by 3 a.m. and the cycle starts all over again.

Chapter 5

Chronic Pain/Treatment

3-27-91 A young man of 38 years old, came in to see me with complaints of numbness of legs and foot pain. The story goes; numbness of left thigh began at least 7 years before, but the heel pain began 1½ years ago followed by numbness in the right thigh. He decided he had better see a doctor. He went to his family doctor, who in turn sent him to a neurologist. Blood tests were done to rule out lead poison and so on. He was given medicines to no avail. He was sent out of town for MRI & EEG, they were normal, then a couple of spinal taps. More medication, and the heel pain worsened. This young man had to rest after standing 5 minutes, so something had to be done for him. He next visited a podiatrist who advised whirl-pool, wrapping the feet for a week then finally fitted him with orthopedic foot wear, which only made the pain worse.

That's when he came to me. There was nothing more to add to what he had already told me. I had the advantage of all the negative studies. This vigorous man had no recall of an injury, no previous injury, no previous back problems, bladder and bowels normal. The hypoasthesia was mainly in the thighs laterally, with both heels tender. The reasoning was correct as far as where the problem was coming from. Treatment must be aimed at his lower back. The needles were inserted, and a series of treatments began. After three treatments, the pain in his feet was gone and slight numbness in thighs only.

On 4-17-91 he said something interesting. He had visited the podiatrist and told him how well he had done with treatments here, and he wanted to return the foot wear and get his money back. After the doctor talked to him for an hour asking all about Acupuncture treatments, the podiatrist gave him his money back, all $250.00.

The patient came back here on 4-24-91 saying he was ready to dance. It was the best he had felt in the past two winters, and was ready to cut hay! The foot pain was only minimal, only felt it towards evening. Treatments were the same, aiming at the lower back and it's nerve distribution. A few more treatments should do it. As this problem clears, he remembered a ski accident years back when he hurt his shoulder. Now that the busy season was about over, and hunting was about to start, he came back for a very localized pain in the right heel. He remained very active, but walking or hunting made it worse. Feet had done well with no relapse. The numbness of the lateral thigh persisted, more to the left. Exam. showed marked tenderness on medial aspect and bottom of right heel; likely a spur formation. Rest of exam negative. 10-10-91; Located, treated spur, much better. The heel was no longer tender, and thighs less numb. As of 10-22-91 he remains asymptomatic.

11-18-85 A young man of 34 years came to see me complaining of lower back pain for about four weeks after trimming a hedge and later changing a tire. The pain radiated down his left extremities. I treated him 3 times.

2-4-91 Severe lower back pain radiating to left leg, and aggravated by cough for a week. No clear accidents. He had just come back from vacation in Banf Canada. The massage sessions while there only worsened the pain. He went to emergency room and was given Robaxisal. Here, he was bent over in agony just trying to move himself around. "Feeling like an old man," he said. Physical findings limited to back, which was tender and tight. Treatment was scheduled for epidural block along with Acupuncture.

On 2-5-91 he was still in pain. He was very worried, because his brother had lumbar laminectomy last year. An MRI was ordered. Report; "Small left paramidline disc herniation at the L5-S1 causing mild to moderate impingement of the left S1 nerve root".

2-6-91 Much better. Walking straight and loosened up, but left sciatica persisted. Discussion of the choice of surgery versus Acupuncture, the benefit and harm of either procedure. MRI findings alone would not be a determinant for surgery. We had to look at the patient's progress. No urgency at this time, so patient decided to continue acupuncture for a while, treatment same as 2-4-91.

2-11-91 Much better. Loosening up and sleeping better.

2-13-91 Continued to improve; similar treatment.

2-19-91 No pain for four days, and he is walking and sitting. Uncomfortable riding in the car.

2-25-91 Woke up stiff from sleeping crooked on couch. No radiation of pain in legs.

2-27-91 Continues to improve; minor spasm of right side.

3-4 & 3-6-91 Minor pain only. No real problem. He will return as needed.

Follow up: 8-92 Continues to do well. I saw him recently in a local restaurant. He said, "Hi, Doc. I feel great, I'm doing my back exercise."

Chapter 6

Case Histories

Organ associated symptoms and signs are shared with western medicine for intensive study and simple cure; diet and drugs, surgery or Acupuncture. Symptoms are viewed by EM from the angles of "Full and void, hot and cold, interior and exterior, Yin and Yang." The treatment has been said to expel the full, and replenish the void. Are drugs less mysterious than needles? You decide.

Case history: A lady came into my office in my early days of allergy practice who had been having allergy problems for fifteen years. She felt so bad, she could not go outdoors and all the screened windows had to be kept closed. At the time of her visit she was using some experimental tongue drops without much success. I suggested she might try Acupuncture, and she agreed to try. After a few treatments she was able to spend three hours in a local park without allergy symptoms. The following summer she came back to see me, stating she could now smell trees and flowers, which she had not been able to do in years. Now, five years later, she is symptom free and enjoying life.

Case 2: A lady of 54 years came in with a Hay fever type allergy she had had since her High school days. She had gone through tests and shots 3 or 4 times with little help. Allergic to pollen, dust, hay etc. Her symptoms were worse in the spring. She was taking heavy doses of antihistamines and losing a lot of sleep because either her nose was plugged or running. She had to get up and drain her sinuses.

This lady was in good health, but had pain in left side of neck, possibly from lack of sleep. Rx; allergy protocol. She came back three days later for another treatment and told me she had slept through the night for the first time in years, she was able to breathe with no getting up at night to look for tissues. After six more treatments, with continued improvement, she was practically asymptomatic without medication. By the conclusion of treatments, as sleep improved, her neck pain also disappeared.

She came back a year later with "sinus congestion" which I diagnosed as "headache" and treated as such. This was not a relapse of her allergy. Again she recovered fully. No allergy, no neck pain, no headache, with good sleep.

Another case history: A 44-year-old man moved here and wanted me to continue his desensitization program for his hay fever, Asthma and eczema he had on his arms. He had moved to the Northwest five years before only to have his allergies worsen every Spring and Fall. He had been treated for allergies as a boy, then stopped treatment for twenty years or so, until this recent bout. This man was taking Topical Steroids and Asthma medicine, yet with all his medicine, he got worse. I suggested to him maybe Acupuncture might be an alternative. He had never heard of using it, but would think about it.

When he came back from vacation, his allergies were worse and wanted to try Acupuncture. The protocols for allergic rhinitis and asthma were explained to him so treatments were given to control his allergic rhinitis and asthma. Half way through the treatments he showed great improvement. He had full course of eight treatments and was practically out of symptoms without medication. His skin cleared up, he could eat better, and he was getting good sleep.

Different views of medicine tend to sentence patients in different ways. If Western medicine considers allergy and asthma as chronic incurable diseases, which can only be put to rest under continuous suppression, that's one view. If Eastern medicine goes ahead and cures the diseases with no further relapse and requires continued treatment, that forms another view. In this case, patients need not get a life sentence. The facts speak for themselves.

One piece of advice I give to you is, "treat Chinese medicine tenderly." It comes out to play only in a supportive, warm and loving environment. It always plays "hooky" on stressful days. The obsession of Western medicine with ordered step by step linear thinking, shuts off direct access to the incredible power of Eastern medicine. Judgment, threat, and pressure only send it running for cover.

Chapter 7

How Acupuncture Works

Having lost confidence in their National power, Chinese and Japanese governments banned the use of Eastern medicine in China and Japan in the past. Now under the name of, "standard of care", set up by the new oppressive government under the cover of "experimental medicine," to refuse payment by insurance companies, so the only option left for Eastern medicine is to play Western medicine games. This leads fragile physicians to practice mediocre medicine.

How can you blend the two? It is not a question of which is more effective, each has it's own place and merit.

To treat an addiction by decraving is certainly more logical than to modify the behavior. It is good to recognize the strength of each party. By studying Western medicine and realizing the scientific principle, this means, you have to study both WM and EM. You have to get into both and get out of both, then you can practice medicine through the fusion of knowledge and wisdom. One cannot argue with success, when patients do well, everyone is happy.

It is with the understanding of our incomplete lack of knowledge we try to theorize the effect of Acupuncture treatment, to sort out how and why it works so well. We may call Acuology the study of Acupuncture, the modern and the Ancient. We will borrow knowledge from Western medicine from time to time to help us out.

Case history: A three-year-old boy with Right facial palsy resulting from a fall against a low table, was brought in to see me after treatments in California failed. He was a well developed little boy for his age. The only deficit was complete right peripheral facial palsy, likely due to trauma. Treatment was given, but he had some trouble with the needles and screamed a lot, not because they hurt, but he was frightened. Three more treatments were given, now right eye closes. Several more treatments were given, and he had full recovery.

Case history: This five-year-old girl was brought in to see if there was help for her nose bleeds, which she had been having for two years. She had been taken to emergency room for care. After four treatments here, no more nose bleeds.

What can we expect to happen from Acupuncture treatment? How can it work? How does it work? It is like asking how does internal medicine work. Despite that kind of question, you swallow all kinds of pills without knowing if they will work.

For five thousand years, the explanations have been metaphysical. Only in the last 100 years or so, along with the advent of modern medicine, we are able to set our eyes on the horizon of physical body and mind. To answer the question concisely, I should start with the way I approach Acupuncture.

This is the usual course of events; someone has a problem, and Acupuncture happens to solve it, even though other modalities fail to do so. Gradually more data about Acupuncturables are accumulated, then a few questions arise: How does it work? What actually happens when the needles are inserted? Is there any medicine in the needles? Why can a plain needle take effect this way? It works through the fine tuning of YIN and YANG, of "Qi (Chi) or, Breath of life." YIN and Yang are in constant change, due to the fact, Normal Qi of Lifebreath within us and Noxious Qi without, are constantly in contact. The FIRE, when harmony waxes, disharmony wanes; when order deteriorates, disorder begins. Restore the system back to order and enjoy harmony and health. The WIND, causes the waterwaves and also causes headache tempest. The rain floods the river, also causes aches and pains in the body.

To set the fire on the Heart or to blow Wind from the Liver may sound as good as an irritable uterus causing hysteria or madness. Hit by the Wind is, Apoplexy, like a fallen tree. Hurt by the Wind, is to catch a cold. The Noxious Qi known to men are, Wind, Fire, Damp, Cold, and Dry. Are they infectious agents? Emotions too are noxious when they are in excess. Can one appeal to the hypothalamus for sexual desire, consult the limbic system for anxiety, etc? Yin Serene and Yang Screen.

"Does it Hurt?" "I don't feel a thing, do you?" No one has run away from the needles yet. I have treated children as young as three years, four, five, six, seven and up.

"When was Acupuncture invented"? Who started to do it first"? "It took me one day to learn, after that, it has been all practice." We learn the basics in school, then you practice and learn. Actually, we read books written two thousand years ago and it still applies today. Human suffering and pain haven't changed much. Only their names change. The study of western medicine only reinforces the need for Acupuncture. "Does it work the same for everyone, in every disease?"

Acupuncture can be mysterious. The thought of using plain needles for treatment is hard to understand. How in the world anyone would think of poking many needles into someone would or could cure such a variety of conditions, is strange. Needles are enchanting, and send you a feeling of something "yonder".

It's effectiveness only enhances the mystery. Stop smoking program has taken care of thousands of people. So has allergy protocol. Cure of headache, neck and shoulder pain became common knowledge. Stress complex is relieved, and more recent, chronic fatigue syndrome becomes curable. All these are done with needles alone, after every "organic" condition has been excluded, and many modalities of treatment failed. "Why is it so effective yet so mysterious?"

How do you know twirling the needle ten times to the right will expel the Noxious Breath, and twirling the needle ten times to the left, will replenish the deficient Normal Breath? Ritual? maybe. How about this; rapid insertion, and slow withdrawal of needle is to expel the saturated Noxious Breath, and the slow insertion with rapid withdrawal of needle is to replenish the Normal Breath? In the latter event, the needle wound is to be covered with the thumb for 30 seconds. Mysterious? Electromagnetic? Who knows?

The depth of needles varies with the seasons. Skin deep in the Spring, subcutaneous tissue in the Summer, Muscle in the Fall, bone and sinew in the Winter.

Organ associated symptoms and signs are shared with western medicine for intensive study and simple cure.

The connection between the mind and organ is by way of Acuflows. The Acuflows flow extensively into the extremities, but eventually get back to the centers. There are five centers. Each kind of Acuflow is connected to it's own center: roughly, assigned to the kidney, is addiction. Two sides of the coin are, Sex and Will. The center of addiction is located in the midbrain. Assigned to the liver, is Behavior. Two sides of emotion are, Love and Hate. The center of Behavior is in Limbic system. Assigned to Heart, is

Conscience. Two sides of Conscience are, Right and Wrong. The center is in the Frontal lobe. Assigned to Spleen, is function of Digestion. The two sides of Digestion are, Health and Disease. The center is in the Motor area. Assigned to Lung, is Environ, way of Exercise. Two sides of Environ are Heaven and Earth. The center is in the sensory area. The sixth area in the brain is the Pons, or bridge. This area concerns the fine tuning of the above five areas by connecting to, Attention, Memory, Anxiety, Tremmer, etc.

Will we see how this system works in acuology? Why does it work? The answer is, no one knows. It is a complete mystery why the human mind should be able to understand anything about the Universe, or microcosms, the body.

All this difference began when God created man of left, and woman of right after His own image. The difference of medicines may just be like man and woman. One is life-support and the other is, life-nurturing. Are two hemispheres right and left brains, really symmetrical? Is this the basis of acucology principle by which it states, "treat the man from the right, and the feminine from the left"?

All at once synthetic process of pattern recognition. We have an extraordinary, miraculous capacity to perceive and process patterns and make them work. It is rather like telling time by looking at an analog clock face instead of reading the digital watch numbers. One picture is worth a thousand words, but a living being is worth a thousand pictures.

A three-year-old came to see me on December 12, 1991 because of urinary frequency at every 15 minutes since November 28. It only happened during the daytime, seldom at night. He had been always in good general health, only recently he had hay fever type of symptoms and sinus infection, and went through allergy test on 11-6-91 by a pediatric allergist. He was then given guafed, beconase and ceclor; family was advised to remove carpet, to wipe mattress with allergy control solution for a month.

He was brought to his pediatrician on 12-2-91, a normal IVP. He was told to stop milk for a week. Yet urinary frequency persisted. What could be done for him? It was then the grandparent called me up and told me about him. She practically told me, "Do something!" Of course, I was hesitant. A 3-year-old boy?

On 12-12-91, the parents brought in detail account of his frequency record: time and amount, up to date. Only a few mililiter each time. But by the grace of God and courage of the parents, he recived acupuncture treatment. After 2 applications, he was going every 4 hours or so. We quit at 4 sessions without further relapse. He screamed and flounced some, but we still remained good friends. When I told the parents that the cause could well be stress, which I treated him for, they looked at each other with a "Hm."

A follow up through the grandparent in September 1992 stated that he continued to do well. The pediatrician was "scientific" enough to retest the antibiotic to see if the urinary frequency could be reintroduced. But it did not occur.

Surprise. Insurance company asked for "medical necessity of acupuncture!"

In December 1991, a 44-year-old male came with a diagnosis of "BHPN" (benign horizontal positional nystagmus), given by a regional University Hospital after extensive studies, including imaging of the inner ears. He had been born with "little rocks" missing in the vestibular tubules of his right ear. This congenital condition has caused the vertigo since birth. He could not drive because of spinning with a simple head swing. He would fall all over in dark places. By mid January of 1992, after 7 sessions of acupuncture treatment, he was able to stand with his eyes closed. "Now that he can stand on his feet, we will get married," said his girl friend.

Chapter 8

Health Care

There are at least two types of people who fall between the cracks of health care. One is obviously financial. If you have no insurance, you can hardly afford it. A few visits and a few tests cost you a bundle. If you have to go into hospital, you had better be prepared, as you will be carefully dissected in detailed billings. When Medicare, welfare, state industrial and some arrogant private insurance companies electively pay, not for certain simpler and more effective affirmative procedures such as Acupuncture, yet pay for all those negative studies, THAT is another story. Patients just try not to come for a more effective mode of treatment they can't pay for, when they do have insurance, who WILL NOT pay for it. Fortunately most private insurance companies will pay for Acupuncture, or at least part of it.

People on Medicare; this form of treatment is treated as "medically unnecessary". Ironically, the denial from Medicare is required for private co-pay insurance to process the claim. This is beside the point.

Another kind of falling between the cracks is, those patients who have been sent to every big clinic in the country without satisfactory solutions. When the tests and machines do not tell some kind of diagnosis, or when the diagnosis is made but no effective treatment can be offered, patients fall in the crack between the doctors and high tech machines. You are on your own. What can you do in this case?

The second type is more intriguing because those cases are being helped here with Acupuncture. These patients fall in the cracks. They start to look around for "unproven" methods of treatment. This of course is taking a greater risk. People go to Mexico for, Laetrel, go to the Philippines for knifeless surgery, and go to pain clinics for Holistic management. Well, Acupuncture has been little known to the common westerners. It has been very effective in many different conditions. One problem is, it is hard to understand in modern terms. Another problem is, everybody seems to do it differently, thus achieving different results. We sure need some kind of "standard of care" here.

Acupuncture has been practiced in certain parts of the world at least 5000 years, and has survived the test of time. It has always been for the people. How much longer do you want to wait and see?

12-01-89

RE: NOTICE TO PHYSICIANS FOR NON-ASSIGNED SERVICES WHICH HAVE BEEN DETERMINED TO BE MEDICALLY UNNECESSARY

I-YEN YANG MD:

Under Section 1842(1) of the *Social Security Act*, a nonparticipating physician who provides services on an unassigned basis which are determined to be unreasonable and medically unnecessary under Section 1862(a)(1) is not permitted to bill the beneficiary for these services.

Please refer to the attached listing of services determined to be not medically necessary.

Explanation #1—Advance Notice Submitted Prior to Initial Determination:

> The service identified has been denied or payment has been made to the patient for a less extensive service because information furnished did not substantiate the need for the service provided. Since you informed the beneficiary prior to furnishing the service that Medicare was likely to deny payment and the beneficiary agreed to pay, the beneficiary is liable for the service provided.

Explanation #2—Advance Notice Not Submitted:

The service had been denied or payment has been made to the patient for the less extensive service because the information furnished did not substantiate the need for the service provided. If you have collected for the denied service or an amount that exceeds your Maximum Allowable Actual Charge (MAAC) for the less extensive service, the law requires you to refund that amount to the patient withing 30 days of receiving this notice. The law permits exceptions to this refund requirement in only two cases:

1. If you did not know, and could not have been reasonably expected to know, that Medicare would not pay for this service; or

2. If you notified the beneficiary before providing the service that you believed that Medicare was likely to deny the service and the beneficiary agreed to pay for the service.

If you come within either of these exceptions, or if you believe the carrier was wrong in its determination that Medicare does not pay for this service, if you should request a review of this determination by the carrier within 30 days of receiving this notice. Your request for review should include any additional information necessary to support your position.

If you request a review within this 30-day period, you may delay refunding the amount to the beneficiary until you receive the results of the review. If the determination on review is favorable to you, then you do not have to make any refund. If, however, the review is unfavorable, the law specifies that you must make the refund within 15 days of receiving the unfavorable review decision.

The law also permits you to request a review of the determination at any time within six months of receiving this notice. A review requested after the 30-day period does not permit you to delay making the refund. Regardless of when a review is requested, the patient will be notifie that you have requested a review and will receive a copy of the review determination.

The patient has received a separate notice of this denial decision. The notice advises that he or she may be entitled to a refund of any amounts paid, if you should have known that Medicare would not pay and you did not tell him or her. It also instructs the patient to contact your office if he or she does not hear anything about the refund within 30 days.

The law specifies that physicians who knowingly and willfully fail to make appropriate refunds may be subject to Civil Money Penalties and/or exclusion from the Medicare program. If you have any questions about this notice, please contact us at the phone number shown on the attached list.

Medicare Department

Chapter 9

Smoking/Addictions

SMOKING: Bad news! Don't think I am going to lecture you on smoking, because you all know the do's and don'ts of it, and I don't think there are many do's around. Doctor Yang has already expressed HIS opinions and views on the subject. He is a kind and caring doctor, but he has a way of letting you know of his displeasure of you (me) smoking. He has never told me outright that I smelled awful, but as that old Chinese saying goes, "A picture is worth a thousand words", he might as well say, "you stink, stop smoking".

Doctor Yang has treated thousands of patients with Acupuncture to stop smoking, with great success. It has been one of the most popular programs. One or two applications and the majority of smokers feel like they had never smoked before. With the realization of the mechanics of addiction, they never smoke again, but so help me, I have not been one of them. He must be the YANG of YIN & YANG, and I must be the YIN. He is such a quiet mellow man, but with a sense of humor, and I am the one who flits along like a butterfly with nowhere to light, and seem to look at life as a gift, just to enjoy, with no regrets. One day recently, I sat still long enough to realize, I don't have to stop smoking for doctors' sake just so I don't hurt his feelings, I have to stop smoking because it is killing me. Many times I have been told to stop smoking or die, because as mentioned earlier in this book, I was born with Asthma.

In honor of my father for Father's Day 1992, over forty years of smoking has finally come to an end. Both of my parents died of cancer, one aunt, one brother-in-law, one cousin, one grandmother, and too many other family and friends have suffered the agony of cancer and death for me to keep ignoring the fact, smoking kills.

Using "The Patch" and acupuncture, it is going to work this time. Like so many other times I have tried to quit by myself and failed after a period of months, fear and determination (with the help of Acupuncture and the patch) are helping me get through the withdrawal "screemy-meemies".

Yesterday, one week later, a dear friend came over (she usually calls first) and told me her husband had a lung collapse on Father's Day, was rushed to the local hospital, then sent to a hospital up in Yakima, Washington. Her husband is a dear man, and a happy guy most of the time but, this really scared him into thinking he was having a heart attack. A collapsed lung is no picnic. He is home now, but still smoking!! My friend leaned over in her chair pointing her finger at me and said, "I want the name of that doctor of Acupuncture you go to. I'm going to call him for an appointment for, (I'll call him Tom) he is going to stop smoking the way you are doing."

This is the same lady friend who has been trying to get me to stop going for Acupuncture treatments for over a year. Dr. Yang's office is about forty miles from here but, the choice is mine; do I want to be in pain, or be pain free? Do I want to smoke or do I want to be smoke free?

Can you imagine the freedom I feel when going out, or going shopping, or traveling, even just going to the post office, and not having to look for my cigarettes and lighter? Feels like a dog must feel being let off a leash to run and play after being tied up all day. Something like that anyway, and the compliments I have received this week are almost too good to be true. "My, don't you look pretty, what have you done"? Or, "Jan, you look great. You look so rested and peppy". or, "My god, what have you done, do you have a new lover"? Now if the health aspect of not smoking isn't enough for you to want to stop, DIG the comments of your friends, and some cute strangers. Finally had to tell everyone why they thought I looked better. Then they didn't want to believe it was just not smoking, but if there is such a big change in the way others see me, can you imagine the changes going on inside my lungs, and the rest of the body's organs?

I would like to tell you something else you might find hard to believe. You know how most people fear gaining weight when they quit smoking? There have been no hunger pangs, no cravings of any kind with one exception, the desire of a cigarette. I know, you all are thinking, "she will never make it", but you are wrong! Acupuncture and the patch will keep me free of smoking.

Two things I do, (don't laugh) a wide rubber band around my wrist and a box of drinking straws. The rubber band is snapped several times until it hurts and I say "Ouch! That hurts", "better your wrist than your lungs". We who have smoked most of our lives have a habit no one else can understand. Ever hear, "you can stop if you want to"? "Stop smoking, you are stinking up the place"? Many more I am sure. Well, I hold a straw in my fingers like a cig. and breathe deep, then exhale. Sound dumb? It satisfies that hand to mouth habit AND, I am breathing in clean air, not smoke.

We are all different, but no one person can forgo a life long habit without help. It's no easier for me than it will be for you when you make that decision. "No discussion, no debate, but, a decision".

Chapter 10

Pain/Acupuncture

Doctor Yang was reading the first half of this Manuscript and he liked what I had written, but told me I should mention something about, some people do feel pain with Acupuncture out of fear of the needles. And, it does not work for everyone because Acupuncture is not "infallible" his words, not mine. I do know someone it did not work on, because this person had already made up his mind it WAS NOT GOING TO WORK. He had decided before he ever went to have treatments for the pain in his back, it was not going to work. This is true only because he had made up his mind to failure before he ever saw the doctor. To this day he wears a nerve stimulater (the black-box) to block the pain, but it does NOT work. He tried to talk me out of going for treatment twenty two years ago, when I was bedridden and getting around in a wheelchair. He tried to make me believe Acupuncture would not work on me, even though he knew nothing about it. The same Orthopedic Surgeon who did the surgery on his back, after a serious accident, is the one who sent me to a doctor of Acupuncture after western medicine had given up on me being able to walk again. This man who wouldn't give Acupuncture a chance to heal his pain, was my daughter's father. Yes, I was married to a man who would deny me a chance to walk again, so I would be totally dependent on him for everything. God forgive him.

Truly, I forgot one time when Acupuncture DID hurt me. If you have read this far, you might remember in the beginning of the book, I was unable to walk. The legs just did not work after falling down five concrete steps on my tail and hip. There was no feeling in them even after all of the hospital stays. I do remember the specialists sticking pins and running a thing that looked like a pizza-cutter with teeth, up and down my legs, hooking me up to machines to test brain-waves, CAT scans, etc., but no one could fix the part of my back that was injured.

After several trips to the doctor of Acupuncture, and beginning to feel just a wee bit of tingling in my legs, this dear man was giving me a treatment lying down in total relaxation, I felt a sharp stab of pain in my big toe of my left foot. "My god, what was that?" I asked him. He began to laugh and asked, "you felt that?" "Yes, I felt that, you jerk". Then I realized I HAD felt it. That was the first time there had been any feeling in my legs or feet in a long time. We both laughed and I guess I cried a bit, because I KNEW I was going to walk again.

That doctor has a special place in my heart. I hope he is still in this country helping those in need.

Chapter 11

Observance of Pleasure

One day at doctor Yang's office not too long ago, I saw a man in a great struggle to make his legs work with the use of two canes, (the kind that wraps around the arm below the elbow) and the look of frustration and pain on his face made my heart ache, but I knew he had come to the right place.

Last week in Dr. Yang's office, while waiting my turn for treatment, this same man was just coming out from his Acupuncture treatment. I looked up and noticed he was using ONE cane, his legs were moving better, but the look on his face is what intrigued me. He was smiling, somewhat of a weak smile, but a smile just the same. His wife helped him some, but you could tell by his expression he wanted to do it himself. I watched fascinated, because I had seen him twice before in the office, all twisted in pain. Watching him getting into their van, his face strained with effort and probably pain, I felt good to see this man try and then succeed, to do it on his own. By the look on his face, he did too. He had made it on his own, and that is a feeling I know well. Can't help wondering about the man, because I haven't seen him since.

It is a wonder to watch someone like that, and know so many others can be helped with Acupuncture, but are afraid,

"They" can't, and really do not know who or where to ask for help. Then there are others who bask in the sympathy they get by being, helpless. What a waste!

Dr. Yang's update:

So you asked about the man? When he first came to me, he rolled on the floor, where I examined him. After his treatments, he is now managing an appliance store of his own.

Chapter 12

Long Ago and Far Away

Long ago, long before the invention of Acupuncture, the lovers of life had searched and researched the joy of health-maintenance and longevity in respect of natural healing mechanisms of our own bodies.

Two major trends came into being; 1) One horizon rose from the breathing exercise, to acupuncture. Both of them quest the nature of 'QI' (pronounced "chee" as in cheese), or breath. They took great pleasure in Qi Gong, which is, "Breath Maneuver", or conscious breathing, to get in touch with brain power. Acupuncture will not work without Qi in action.

2) Another horizon raised from food to drugs. It never went the way of chemistry or biochemistry. It took the course of metaphysics so it assumes that food and drugs also harbour Qi, and are to be classified according to taste, smell, temperature, etc. It becomes harder to swallow when food and drugs are assigned to be bearers of breath which is guided by smell, and treats the nose. Understandably, this is giving the mechanical world a breath of life.

With the discovery of Antibiotics and the improvement of dietetics and public health, most acute and curables have been taken care of. The weight has been shifted to more chronic and incurables. Thus, we turn to the quest of the nature of Qi Gong and acupuncture.

—C F HUANG TI & YEN TI

The mystery of life and breath is important because, when we quit breathing, we die. No wonder we stress the "Breath of Life". Some call it breath, others call it, Spirit. There is a school in Japan, in which combined both (spirit) Rei and (breath) Ki. Do we become aware of the act of Spiritual-breathing? It is interesting that we aren't usually aware of the act of breathing when we are well, it is only part of our routine. Inhale air in through the nose, larynx, trachea and lungs with the use of our chest muscles and ribs. The command comes from the brain. Breathing is done so insidiously we have to study to find it; we breathe 12-18 times a minute, 23,040 times a day; we sigh every 6 breaths or so, and we only use one quarter of our lung capacity to breathe. The rest of the 7 billion alveoli lie lazy. The lungs blame the muscles for not doing the job. Fact is, muscles are truly underworked. Only 10 percent of the microcirculation in the muscles are at work at any given time, so the rest are just waiting. How about the brain? It is supposed to be in command. That's a good question. There are billions of neurons in the brain, 140 billion to be exact, but we use only about 10 billion. What a waste! What can we do about it?

There is one thing we can do to rectify the situation. We can do a near full lung breathing exercise, or even a whole body breathing exercise by using muscle more extensively, or at least once in awhile. We only need to practice it a few times a day to keep in shape. The whole process of "conscious muscle breathing" (CMB) is done in an orderly fashion, to reinforce the circulation of Qi itself by sequential movement of the back muscles in a state of meditation. Here is the principle; Move the breath consciously and let the breath move the body. In mechanics, this is how it goes;

1) Stand straight with eyes looking forward. Inhale as you lift the Qi from the anus to the top of head;

2) Move the Qi down the neck and upper back; as you keep on inhaling slowly to move

3) Qi down the diaphragm and mid-back;

4) Qi down the lower back and abdomen;

5) Exhale; as you relax.

6) Resting state; now you are in total relaxation.

You will be pleasantly surprised to find these simple exercises will ease the muscle spasms of head and neck, back and legs, so the aches and pains dissipate, or at least you will feel refreshed. Did you feel at ease and the lump in you chest vanish? Don't make a ritual of this when you do it either. Please read on, we are getting closer to the truth.

Chapter 13

No Brain In Chinese Medicine

There was no brain in Chinese medicine. Chinese medicine is so functionally oriented that the brain has been taken for granted, or thought to be in existence as a matter of fact. After you have worked through the central theme of Chinese medicine, you realize that the function of the brain is clearly woven into the organ system. It is safe to say that Chinese medicine is all organs and no brain. Lets take a look at the categories of organs as follows:

a) Yang organs (bowels) gall, stomach, intestine, colon, bladder, trifoci. The bowels are responsible for the passage and excretion of waste.

b) Yin organs (viscera) heart, liver, spleen, lung, kidneys, cardiover. Qi (breath) blood and fluid are stored here.

c) Wonder or Curious organs; brain, marrow, bone vessel, gall bladder, uterus.

d) Special senses, genitalia, hair, skin, muscle, and bone become part of viscera and bowels.

e) Emotions are indwelling in the organs.

As YIN and YANG relationship is carried over to areas in medicine, the concept of YIN and YANG appears in the discussion of organs and Acuflows, physiology and pathology, prevention and treatment.

If we extract the brain from E.M. we can then see how the actual brain functions. Briefly, there are 5 or 6 functional units in the brain:

1) Motor center to direct everything that moves. Obviously muscle is one. Heart, intestines and internal organs also move. Some cells move independent of nerves, and are considered dispatched nerve cells, such as white blood cells. Muscles are balanced by deep senses.

2) Autonomic nerves get involved with the internal organs. The eventual center is the motor center of the brain. For the sake of discussion, it is desirable to separate the two and let the muscular skeletal be one, and internal organs be another unit. The internal organs are simply divided into upper (cardiopulmonary), middle (gastrointestinal) and lower (urogenital) foci: so called Trifoci.

3) Senses and sensory center are another obvious unit. Their centers occupy the back part of the brain.

This 3 parts of the brain and the belongings is commonly known as life science. No doubt this portion of the body is easily subjected to much study. There are three more functional units in the brain, the three oblivions:

4) The hypothalamus with it's hormonal impetus. This is the kidney power in Chinese medicine, where the story of the serpent and temptation is depicted. It is the temple of mystic with incense smoke. Succumb to temptation, and

we become fallen Angels. An overdose is the cause of hyperfunction which includes, compulsion and obsession, cravings and addiction. Trying to understand the pharmacological estrogen dose of breast cancer treatment, is a risky business. acupuncture restores the depleted endorphine, when the addicts are treated.

5) The limbic system and emotion, from love and jealousy. Greek Mythology and psychology lead us to ecstasy in some imaginary world. This is the theater of many dramas. It is where tranquilizers do their work. Tranquilizers such as Valium, seriously interfere with the effect of acupuncture treatment, as they compete with the same receptors in the lymbic system.

6) Frontal lobe is responsible for judgment and conscience. This is where Chinese medicine tends to call the heart of the mind which means, the "Commander of the body". It is not the frontal lobe that says, "thou shall not do this or that", the hypothalamus just ignores the command and says, "go for it". How do we follow what we preach, as we can beat up on anyone from the point of guilt.

This 3 parts of the brain and it's belongings is commonly known as, the study of human nature.

If the 3 parts of the brain and it's belongings is known as the study of human behavior, why are the effects of hormone and unmelinated nerve fibers more lingering and diffuse in nature with some more tenacious than others? We wonder if the brain tumors of William Casey and Atwater have had serious effects on their behavior.

The "Pons" is so named because it is literally a bridge. It is the hub of the above mentioned 6 units of the brain. Anatomy and physiology tell us about the function of reticular formation and later A-10 nerves of this area. These nerves connect to all of the above units, and when under stress, can affect every system by way of this bridge. Every known symptom expresses itself under the situation. The breath exercises confront this area which regulates the sleep as well as wake rhythm, the immune response and well being. Lack of sleep lowers the immune mechanism among other things. It also lowers the stress threshold, allergy causes emotional distress. It is right to say that allergy is emotional from this point of view. Without negative feedback mechanism, the messengers are like ghosts, free to come and go. In some point, creativity breaks through like an open valve, that thin layer of insanity.

A recent twist came from France when Dr. Nogier discovered the inverted ear to be a picture of an embryo, or a projection of the human body. Later Dr. Ang of China pointed out the theory of ECIWO in reference to the acupuncture point. This states that each part of the body is an ultimate embryo in a certain developed stage with full potential. So the hand is a visible part of the brain, the foot a tangible part of the heart. Inside of our bodies is made visible when we open two inverted ears coupled together to make a whole body. This makes the inner space accessible. The ear lobe exposes the brain to the acupuncturists. The folds and creases are corresponding to the gyri of the brain. By knowing these nerve endings relationship to conditions such as stress, allergy, addictions of food and drug, they become treatable. Sounds like a break through, but there are still missing links to be found. We still need biochemical events at the cellular and molecular level to explain the effect of acupuncture. Where are the academicians?

We can read books written 1000 years ago and apply the treatments today. The truth keeps going on forever as long as human beings exist. For example, the Compendium of Acupuncture and Moxibustin by, Yang JuJou during the Ming Dynasty, gave a good overview of the general practice of acupuncture.

Chapter 14

Stress

In many books of classic E.M., we find the detailed symptoms, descriptions of symptoms and their treatment. It takes symptoms, regardless of causes, as final common pathways of human suffering, which have not changed through the ages. The Acupoint well defined to be at the nerve endings, is the point where the symptoms are reduced to one. This is like looking at the world through a grain of sand. The location of tenderness, nodule, color change, and the inflammation, where are they pointing? Are they a local problem or an internal disorder? This makes diagnosis less important. What does it mean when we say, "sinus headache", or migraine? Is it merely a headache, an allergy, or part of stress syndrome? So many questions, do we have the answers? The acupoint signals the status of health. It is up to us to find the meaning of it. The emphasis of Surprise Acuflows and their application is not only intriguing, but heart-warming. The idea of mental effect of Wellspring Acupoint, came through these teachings.

As each birth is a hope for new beginnings, so is each breath a renewal of hope. Limited knowledge ought not force us to the mystic and the dark ages. We need to open up and breathe freely with relish.

I was amused when a patient showed me an article in which acupuncture was thought of as, "a possible mystical technique of the new-age movement". I also chuckled when a patient disappeared after I mentioned the Holy Spirit could play a big part in the cure. "What is known is knowledge, what is unknown is Divine". With limited knowledge of biology, the "Ancient Ones", tended to take a global view of disease. They stated, "it is easier to practice than to understand". Is that why we are practitioners?

The ancient scholars have concluded, there were three treasures in human beings; The mind, the body and the organ. These are the areas we can work on and strengthen through "QI" or breath. The so called normal Qi is the idea of healthy hematology and immunology at their best. If we eat sensibly and exercise, try CMB, then we can ward off our short comings, and we can live a better lifestyle. To be at peace with ourselves, without fear of noxious Qi or agents that attack the human body from any point of view, good or bad and keep the battle ground outside our bodies so it does not enter our system, then we should find new found health.

The "beast" of the kidney which is treated by the acupoint of the ears, sword of the liver, which eyes can watch it, legality of the heart for the tongue to serve it, famine of the spleen with the mouth, pest of the lung by the nose. Once we get entangled with noxious "Qi" and the battle ground does establish itself in our bodies, symptoms are inevitable. Acupuncture continues to restore the internal organs and alleviate aches and pains.

Different views of medicine tend to sentence patients in different ways. If western medicine considers allergies and asthma as chronic incurable diseases which can only be put to rest under continuous suppression, that is one view point. If eastern medicine goes ahead and cures the diseases with no further relapse and requires no continuous treatment, that forms another view. In this case, patients need not get a life sentence. The facts speak for themselves. I would like to discuss some similar problems in common. Let me start with a condition called, "Chronic Fatigue Syndrome". (CFS) is a complex of symptoms which usually come on all at once. As I have seen more and more cases of similar complaints, irrespective of different causes, I began to see some patients with an illness, not necessarily a disease.

The causes are usually some sort of stress, physical or mental. Most stress is like the weather, nothing one can do about it. The idea begins to make sense when we see how Chinese medicine uses changes in the weather as analogy of human ailments, both as, cause and effect. The wind can cause a head cold, the "wind" also originates from the liver to cause convulsions. The fire can cause febrile illness, the "fire" also originates from the heart to cause canker sores.

Stress may include such things as, human nature, warfare, government, famine and pestilence. A past history of, child abuse, failing marriage, sickness in the family or oneself, child birth, business disaster or state of mind, can all play a part of stress. This makes history taking of the patient very important. Some times it may sound like gossiping, but it can be essential in helping to pinpoint the cause of stress.

Although the causes of stress may vary, the symptoms are so alike that the patients start to blend together. I don't mean their faces, but their sufferings. Due to the stress, the nervous system loses the balance of central fine tuning mechanism, which is likely in the reticular formation. All aspects of negative feedback go to pot. The patient is not only emotionally depressed, but jittery and shaky. Physically, multi-organ symptoms may appear in time. Palpitations, chest pain, abdominal distress, irritable bowels, to name a few. As insomnia progresses, energy dwindles. Taught nerves and tense muscles are the result of aches and pains in all areas; neck and shoulder, back and legs being the most prominent. A stiff neck is often accompanied by headache, which tends to affect the eyes and other senses. It could be called neck and back sprain or myofacia pain syndrome. In females, this complex may be called P.M.S.

Allergies become worse which make the patient more vulnerable to infection. Even the skin is affected. Minor skin infection and seborrhea dermatitis are common. It eventually affects the concentration and memory. Not only are the symptoms alike, but the course of illness and treatment they have to go through are more or less identical. The physical findings are generally scanty in spite of a multitude of complaints. The laboratory studies are predictably negative. The EB virus and yeast connection are red herrings. X-rays of neck and back are negative, with occasional incidental findings of degenerative changes. M.R.I. of head shows nothing wrong. After a prolonged course of treatments, at last they are often told that nothing more could be done, and there was nothing wrong physically to start with. This is told to patients with a straight face, in spite of all their physical symptoms. The patients usually end up being put on analgesics, antidepressants, tranquilizers, sleeping pills, and so forth. Since the inner force and outer environs are hard to change, just like the weather, it is essential for oneself to build up the immune system to ward off the stresses and be in harmony. In other words, it is hard to change the stress in your life, as there will always be stress of some kind or another, but one can learn to cope and make the best of it.

Nothing is so big that one can't handle it, Heaven won't fall down, it's not the end of the world. All of this is easier said than done, I know. You have tried religion, art, logistics, nutrition, exercise, but you have only become more tired and frustrated. Makes you wonder, doesn't it?

It is not unusual for this chronic fatigue syndrom to go on for years unless it is treated, and treated properly. People come to see me as a last resort, after western medicine has failed them. If they happen to drop in, they are fortunate, because if they run around in this vicious circle, the average duration of their illness before they come here, is five years. Some of them have suffered 8 to 15 years. It becomes so frustrating, many patients quit planning for their future.

Can acupuncture really help? Most likely. My experience with this particular symptom complex has been excellent. The amazing part is, that all the symptoms disappear at once as the treatment proceeds, just like they have appeared all at once in the beginning. Only because of the favorable responses, I began to figure out retrospectively how this procedure is supposed to work.

By placing needles in certain acupoints, patient's perspectives are restored, and conflicts are lessened so the physical symptoms are abated. It works through the negative feedback system, to let the feedback mechanism get back in gear.

Where does this put Ms. L.L.? I shall answer your questions as follows:

1) She is disabled according to either of your definitions. She has been working around her fatigue, rather than counting on her energy. This is typical of, Chronic Fatigue Syndrome;

2) She is not able to perform her duty;

3) The natural course of CFS is unpredictable, but it is usually a prolonged case. My experience with this type of condition is, the patient is willing but the energy is wanting. The prognosis is guarded at best;

4) Fatigue itself prevents her from returning to work. My outline of the condition above should give you some insight;

5) No medication has shown cure of this ailment. Most people have tried, antidepressants, anti-inflamatories, and tranquilizers. The most recent report from NIH needs to be investigated. My own experience with acupuncture in treating a few dozen cases gives better than 90% for full recovery in one to six months.

Chapter 15

Illustrations

The Meridians of Acupuncture: The Acuflows and How They Affect the Whole Body

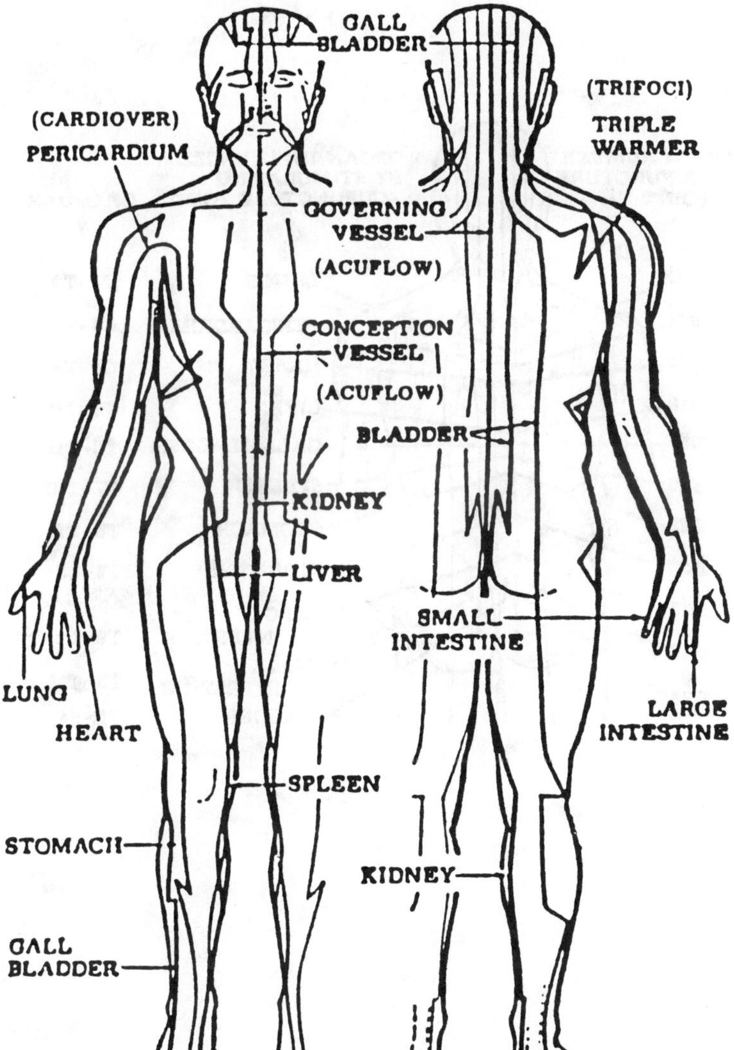

Acupuncture Points

Some of the acupuncture points, particularly on the back that have an effect on a specific organ, are in the appropriate Acupoints.

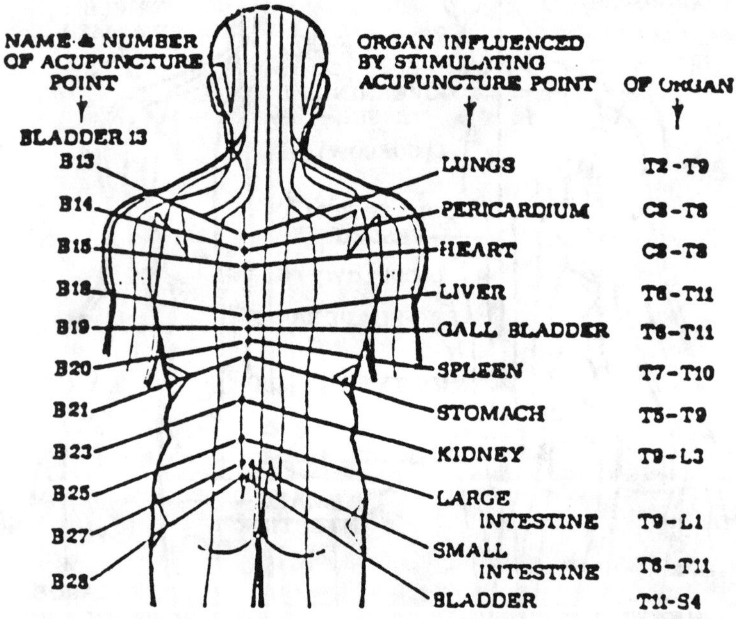

On page thirteen, I asked you to try to imagine a round pie shaped picture in your mind so you would know which organs are doing what in your body, and at what time. I decided to show you what I mean. Hope this helps make you more aware of how our bodies work, and the job they are doing. I find this fascinating.

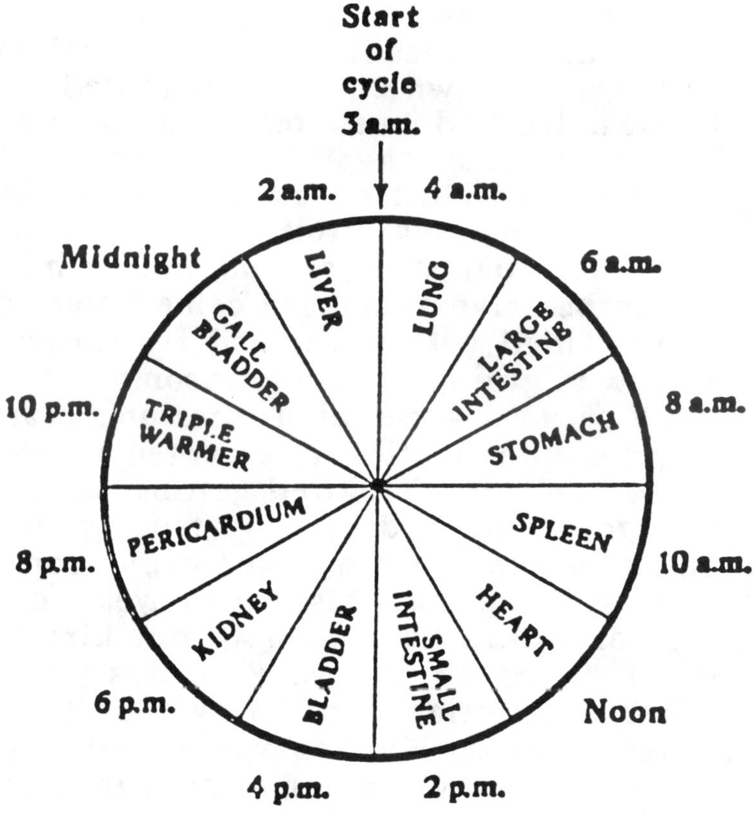

Even while we sleep, our internal organs are working for us.

Chapter 16

More Case Histories

Case #1: A 37-year-old male; CFS. This man has had "Chronic Fatigue Syndrome" for three and a half years. It started with intense "spin" without warning. He began to fall to the left and backwards, with this sensation never leaving him, and leaving him with a right sided earache which he attributed to allergies. He had been tested by a local allergist who later gave him a diagnosis of CFS. After exhausting all tests here, he was sent to regional multispecialty clinic where the prognosis was guarded, it may last another five years. He came home in despair, filled with anger and frustration. Chronic migraine, allergy, insomnia and fatigue became worse. Sinus pressure, heart burn, and constipation interrupted by the urge to "go". He felt tired getting up and tired going to bed. Exhausted by ten o'clock in the morning, he would come home so drug out his seven year old daughter would have to help put him to bed on the couch. At work he was given further restrictions so he wouldn't be further injured. He was very careful at work not to show any emotional impact, (so no psychological needs would be suggested). He had gained 35 pounds due to inactivity. Physical exams were essentially negative except that he was a husky man who appeared to be tired and frustrated. This man could not remember some of the events through the course of the illness, so his wife had to fill in the blanks.

After eleven Acupuncture treatments he was feeling wonderful and going strong. He had torn down a building to build a garage. A year later there was a relapse of the right ear problem. The ear had been treated for infection several months before when he felt pain and thickness in the ear. He also began to lose his balance which gradually got worse. His insomnia returned temporarily from being up-tight and frustrated. Family doctor gave him decongestants which helped the balance problem, but gave him the shakes and palpitations. The imbalance had been a steady state with episodic aggravations of vertigo, often evoked by a moving target or high pressure chambers at work. Three years had passed, there wasn't any headache, sneezing, itchy eyes and no wheezing. This patient has made good progress. He probably never had CFS. It has been reduced to simple vertigo of inner ear origin which rarely bothers him any more.

Case #2: This is a 73-year-old lady. In August 1990, she woke at 1 A.M. with neck pain; headache followed. Since then she woke up every morning with ear, jaw and eye pain. She could hardly find any comfortable position. She had no vomiting or nausea. After initial x-rays and failure of muscle relaxant and physical therapy, she had an MRI of head and neck. This came out normal. She had had lumbar disc surgery in 1947.

After a helicopter crash in 1983 when her son died, her backache returned. Her husband died a year and a half later, after the crash. She had since then suffered insomnia. She used alcohol to help her sleep, at least four drinks a night. This lady ate while she was drinking so she gained 35 lbs. She had had a hysterectomy in 1977 for cancer of the uterus. Appearing depressed and anxious, always nervous, I wondered what would be the treatment for her. Could this be a locally treatable condition? After three treatments she continued to do well except for pain in the neck. She also decided she wanted to get rid of 20 pounds. Continued improvement. Now she is telling me about her mother in hospital dying from renal cancer. Her mother, a lady of 89 years, fell, breaking her right hip. Mother has Alzheimer's disease to boot. More treatments for my patient for neck pain. 1-28-91 still having pain in neck. Mother has only one more week to live but continues to live. Patient has pain in neck, insomnia, eating problem, only eating one meal a day. More treatments. She is spending all day at hospital with mother, drinking more at home; tiredness, insomnia, aches and pains, poor memory. Hurts her to drive. You got it, time to treat the STRESS. More treatments for drinking and weight gain. No pain for a week and sleeping without nightmares. Still "Mother sitting" but coping better; minor urge to drink but didn't have one; Rx. weight control protocol; 3-12-91 she has done well. Under control, both with food and drink. Same treatment. Three months since last seen.

6-6-91 One of this lady's neighbors came in for back problem said Virginia has been doing excellent and sends greetings. 12-23-91 Virginia back again with a new problem; Right shoulder pain for two months. Seems, three great-grand children aged, 3, 5, and 11 "dropped in" for past 4 months. Grandson just got divorced and jobless. She felt tied down, but had to help. No headache, no backache; sleeping well with no desire to drink; has lost 20 pounds so far and kept it off. She is doing yard work and driving, among other things. Another of her neighbors came in and gave me further details of her misfortune; She has another grandson who called her from jail with a drunk-driving charge, wanting her to send money. According to the neighbor the story of the helicopter accident went this way: The helicopter crashed near Mt. St. Helene. She was the least wounded, her husband stayed at a local hospital for a few days. Her son and she were released from hospital after an overnight stay. Soon the son felt pain in his neck at home, which prompted him to visit the family doctor at Moses Lake, who saw a broken neck on the x-rays. He was flown to Seattle and stayed in a straight jacket; followed for another year. After being home, he was in a local Deli for a glass of Coke, which he loved to do. He died instantly when he raised the glass to his mouth to drink, by extending his neck back.

This neighbor who was telling of the crash and the hell the patient was going through, has a hobby of listening to the police scanner. One day he heard, "Walter was hit by a car while crossing the street". "That's Virginia's husband!" Seems Walter often took walks since the helicopter accident. "Didn't expect him to go this way." The helpful neighbor also mentioned Virginia's mother, who finally died after a long period of agony. "Oh, by the way, she has a brother who has Alzheimer's disease". Oh! the art of history taking is hard to master!

At the time of her last visit she lamented, "I wish I had never told my son I would give him the fare for the helicopter ride. He expressed the wish to go on the ride, and I gave him the money."

Writer's note;

After reading this lady's story, I am reminded of Job, in the Bible. God tested him, but I think this lady has Job beat hands down. I ask the Holy Spirit to lift her burdens! This page ends with a tribute to a lady named, Virginia.

Update: She is now living with 13-year-old great-grand daughter and will stay with her until finish of high school. The grand son finally found a job, took the two younger kids with him, leaving this lovely lady of 76 years to raise the great-grand daughter.

About the Author

M. Jeannette Cunningham was born and bred in southern California where she lived until she knew it was time to get out on her own. She lived the good life as a girl with her parents of upper class Irish, in an exclusive neighborhood.

Even as a child she couldn't understand the bigotry and prejudice of her family and of the people in her immediate neighborhood, so she began to write stories about them to sell to *Reader's Digest*.

"I was a precocious child but kept quiet about my feelings and observations, but kept wondering why, when my grandfather took me with him to visit a friend, who just happened to be black, I was told, 'Don't tell Mama.' Or when he took my sister and I with him to visit his friend, 'Old John' who lived at the dump, the kind man who let us run all over the dump looking for treasures, we were told, 'Don't tell Mama.' Or when Papa went to visit his friend the old Chinese man, who grew wonderful vegetables (and always sent us home with the back seat full of fresh veggies) I was told, 'Don't tell your Mother or Father.' "

At the tender age of nineteen, I set out to find out just what was wrong with these people I was not supposed to speak to or associate with. First going to Stanford University then further north to Cal-Poly, then even further north to Berkley University where I was thrown into a mixture of every race and culture. The end of the rainbow. My life now had purpose and meaning. I was to spend the rest of my youth and adult life helping others to be open minded, being able to see his or her brother or sister of different color, race or life style, as a human heart to be treated tenderly and with care.

As a published author, I have written articles for magazines, a novel which was sold for the movie rights, and a series of books for children, and now this little book. A new series of books about and for children, and two books of poetry as yet unpublished.

About the Co-Author

I-Yen Yang was born in China, where he lived with his parents while going to school. He did his pre-med studies in China, where he received his Medical Doctorate degree.

When Dr. Yang came to the U.S.A. he did internship and Residency at Pittsburgh and Detroit hospitals. Dr. Yang received his fellowship at Cleveland Clinic in Ohio. He then went into practice in the Northwest, where he and his wife bought a home, raised their two children, sent them to school here, and now have a son and daughter studying medicine.

Dr. Yang has many medical specialties and sub-specialties. He is also a doctor of Internal Medicine, Hematology, medical Oncology, Allergy and Immunology.

In 1974 he went back to Beijing China to study the art of Acupuncture, because he knew the mixture of Western Medicine and Eastern Medicine could be of beneficial help to his (and many other) patients of long suffering.

Dr. Yang feels he has healed more people with Acupuncture than all the other specialties and sub-specialties combined.

As a published author, he has had Medical studies published in Taiwan in the *Central Daily*. He has had medical school publications, and was the editor of a magazine in college. He is still a contributing member of a poetry magazine called *The Vineyard Quarterly*.

Dr. Yang has gone back to Taiwan to give tests to Chinese medical students, in Western Medicine.